Wheat Free Diet

The Ultimate Guide to Eating Wheat Free, Losing Your Belly, and Keeping It Off!

By **Natalie Ray**

Disclaimer

This book is a self-help guide that gives reader valuable tips on how better understand the "wheat free diet." This book provides the reader with a better understanding of the diet in hopes of making a difference in the reader's life.

The author of this book is not affiliated with any medical company, nor does the author provide medical treatment advice in any way. The ideas, views, and opinions expressed in this book are those of the author. The author assumes no liability for advice or suggestions offered in this book. The author and publisher of this book and the accompanying materials have used their best efforts in preparing this book. The author and publisher make no representation or warranties with respect to the accuracy, applicability, fitness, or completeness of the contents of this book. The information contained in this book is strictly for informational purposes. Therefore, if you wish to apply ideas contained in this book, you are taking full responsibility for your actions.

Wheat Free Diet: Ultimate Guide to Eating Wheat Free, Losing Your Belly, and Keeping It Off! Copyright © 2013 by **Natalie Ray**. All rights reserved. No part of this book may be reproduced in any form without permission in writing from the author.

Table of Contents

Introduction to "Wheat Free"

A lot has been said and written on one of the most interesting diet topics of today –"The Wheat Belly Diet." But, is it really enough to convince people to eliminate one of their most beloved food items from their diet? After all, this is one food, the advantages of which, they have been learning all their lives; the foundation of the ever-popular food pyramid.

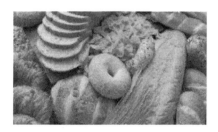

Is it possible that they are missing out on something or perhaps the Wheat Belly Diet isn't for everyone? In this book, I will provide you with a clear understanding of the Wheat Belly Diet, what foods you can eat, what foods you should avoid, and I even provide a few delicious example recipes! Following my book, and following the concept of the "Wheat Belly Diet" can provide you with some amazing, life changing results! Later in this book, I provide you a "before and after' picture of a young lady—you will be amazed by her results! If she can do it, so can YOU!

So what's holding you back? Break down all the barriers, grab your notepad, and let's get started. Be sure to grab your FREE bonus at the end of the book as well!

Overview: Why Turn Against Wheat

Dr. William Davis has recently been seen on many of the leading talk shows and all he focuses on is the new diet rage, known as the 'Wheat Belly Diet.' Now, there are a few corrections that have to be made here, before we can move forward. First of all, Dr. Davis has not tried to create a diet rage, as some people might think (frankly as I thought so too earlier). Instead he is trying diligently to spread the awareness amongst people of how some medical conditions are linked to wheat. The message that he is conveying to the world is not based on some kind of whim, but is in fact only a result of lessons that he has learned through personal experiences.

The phrase 'Wheat Belly Diet' (which is gaining popularity rapidly) is wrong as Dr. Davis doesn't mention the word 'diet' in juxtaposition to Wheat Belly in either of his two books. He does explain the term Wheat Belly and what edible products our diet should consist of. It is more of a lifestyle change forever than an eating regime that has to be followed for short duration to reach a short-term goal.

Dr. Davis, like most other American children, had spent his childhood and college years feasting on ready-made meals, sandwiches, burgers, bagels, pizzas, pies and what not; basically hearty foods in all you can eat patterns.

Consequently, his teenage years and those spent in college, when he should be running around and enjoying the peak of his agility, were spent feeling tired, heavy and sleepy. To battle all these side-effects he upgraded his daily dose of caffeine; but as he grew older he became diabetic like millions of other Americans.

He soon realized that he was constantly advising his diabetic patients to lead a healthy lifestyle and to increase the intake of fresh fruit and vegetables alongside the healthy whole grains and yet was himself not practicing any of it. Yet with a diet change he still felt fuller than he desired and there was no change in his blood sugar levels. However, he did comprehend that in days where he had a wheat-free breakfast, he felt more agile and more awake. And this is where he experimented with both organic wheat meal and wheat-free meal. To his surprise, Dr. Davis discovered that even while consuming the healthy grains his sugar level sky-rocketed and when he substituted it with a wheat free option, it only climbed within a normalcy range. As an added advantage he found himself to be more active and full of zip. Upon following the new eating regime, he ended up losing the extra weight around his belly (that he was carrying around for a long time) and cured his diabetes.

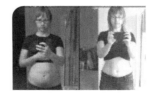

Therefore, as part of his treatment he advised his diabetic patients to do the same and within months, all of his patients started showing the same results – they had lost as much as 20 – 40 pounds and their diabetes was gone. However, up until now he had thought that wheat was the culprit causing the blood sugar levels to rise and therefore it needed to go. While his patients shared their experiences, they also shared other changes that they had been experiencing: decreased or vanished joint pain, some were happy to reveal that their irritable bowel syndrome has gone or that they are also cured of asthma. And soon he was unable to put aside such constant comments and had to wonder about the harmful elements contained inside the wheat that lead to so many other health issues.

Harmful Components of Wheat

This is how the certified preventive cardiologist, took it upon himself to find out more about wheat and its constituents. In his book, Dr. Davis compares wheat to a loyal spouse who's true and unfaithful intentions are unfolded; because this is exactly how dear we hold wheat to ourselves.

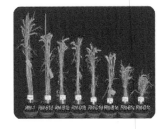

Through his discovery about the history of the new wheat, he exposed many lurking dangers present inside this almost-artificial and cruel product. The first thing that he ascertained was that the present wheat is not comparable to what was eaten in the days of our grandparents or even when our parents were young. The wheat, and its various kinds, available to the masses is only a product which has resulted from continuous genetic alteration of wheat genes in order to come up with a better yielding crop; something that could yield more grain in a given square area. The original long stalk of wheat is now reduced to a mere 18-inch crop. The sad part is that while scientists and geneticists were busy altering the genes with good intentions they overlooked the most vital aspect of testing on animals or on humans.

Dr. Davis revealed that the following extremely destructive elements are present in wheat that cause a multitude of common complaints in our body; while some of these are troubling (laziness, anxiety, mind fogging), others are really serious like asthma, bowel disorders, rheumatoid arthritis, diabetes and heart diseases. My first book Wheat Belly Diet: Ultimate Guide to Losing Your Wheat Belly and Feeling Amazing! contains a detailed account of the harmful substances in wheat; my second book (a cookbook with wheat-free recipes) also mentions them. However for those who haven't, here is a brief description of those harmful elements.

- **Amylopectin A:** Amylopectin A is one of the complex carbohydrates present in wheat that makes it more harmful than other carbs like rice. This is the substance that causes the sudden upsurge in blood sugar levels as it is easily absorbed in the body through organ linings.

Carbohydrates in rice do not get absorbed as easily and therefore we don't get that high after eating rice and other such carbs. This sudden sugar high comes crashing down moments later and we are all too familiar with this feeling. When our body develops a craving, we usually look for something to snack upon from the refrigerator; maybe it is the leftover pizza slice from last night or a quick sandwich with a friendly serving of some sort of spread or leftover cooked meat in between. After snacking, we usually find ourselves to be full of energy abruptly; this is actually the sugar high that we are experiencing which makes us even more lethargic later on. Dr. Davis explains that eating two slices of bread is equivalent to consuming 6 teaspoons of table sugar or a small candy bar.

- **Gliadin:** Another culprit found in wheat is Gliadin. It is a kind of protein in wheat that has the ability to breakdown into smaller proteins or polypeptides and then reaches to a specific area in our brain through blood. The morphine receptors that it attacks, are responsible for building up the feeling of pleasure inside us; for instance the feeling that overcomes us when we bite into a luscious chocolate bar. And this is the reason that we have an undying urge to keep snacking on something 'wheaty' and not on other stuff like fruits and vegetables. Gliadin is also responsible for getting us hooked on the various wheat products in a similar way like we get addicted to caffeine or alcohol. Hence when we plan on leaving it or actually start cutting it out of our lives, we feel the separation anxiety and it might even lead to slight depression. It is therefore advised to reduce its intake slowly at first and then just go 'cold turkey' as Dr. Davis puts it.

- **Lectins:** Then we have the Lectins which are perhaps some of the most potentially dangerous substances present inside wheat. These are also smaller proteins but ones that have the ability to unlock the proteins in the intestine lining so that they can creep inside the blood. The wall lining present in the intestine is there to prevent the absorption of harmful substances inside the body and only allows the inclusion of beneficial nutrients into the blood so they can be utilised. When the Lectins creep into our system, they can virtually reach any part of the body becoming the root cause of auto-immune diseases like heart diseases, arthritis and diabetes. And therefore, Dr. Davis discovered that upon removing wheat out of their diets, his patients were cured from these different diseases.

Now how do we link these ills of wheat with a hanging belly, he calls Wheat Belly. The Amylopectin A and the Gliadin both act in a way that it induces an increased appetite. So even if we were to argue that people in the old days also consumed wheat but were not generally obese, was because they ate the original 14-chromosome wheat what has now been genetically altered with other kinds of wild grasses to yield a 42-chromosome wheat crop that has been nurtured by nitrate fertilizers.

Dr. Davis has done ample amounts of research on the harmful effects of consuming modern-day wheat and has discovered that appetites of people has increased a lot since the olden days and now they roughly consume around 400 more calories per day for every day of the year leading to obesity and hanging weight around the belly.

Dieters have the knack of automatically cutting out all sorts of fat from their diet, in order to prevent the excessive weight gain. However, according to Dr. Davis, we don't need to cut down on fats (healthy ones) or on the different dairy products; all that is required is eliminating the wheat from our kitchen and our pantries.

The one thing that people need to understand is that eating fat does not make fat in the body. It is all the unused calories which we have consumed during the day along with the toxins that are absorbed within the body which lead to excessive inches around the belly, thighs, hips and arms. So everything and anything that our body thinks is in an excess, goes down the storage path in the shape of fats.

Therefore, those who eat the wheat-carbs in excess, suffer from a lot of health problems. These conditions can be wide ranging but thankfully Dr. Davis says that all these conditions can now not only be prevented but can be reversed as well. So if that is true, (and it is, because many of his patients have revealed it with their own individual experiences), it would be wondrous to follow a healthy eating routine that does not involve the intake of strong and harmful medicines and which leads to complete health.

What to Eat and What NOT to Eat!

There is a strong argument prevailing that if you cut out the wheat from your diet, then you miss out on the fibres that are needed for a healthy digestive system too. The statement seems logical, but Dr. Davis believes that thousands of years ago, when man first started to roam the earth, his diet was not based on carbs gained from wheat and other grains. In fact, man relied on meat and other direct sources of food, like vegetables and fruits, for energy. It is when man included wheat into his diet that things started to go wrong for him.

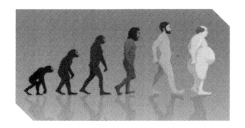

The man of earlier times was certainly more agile and was able to live a long and healthy life. The coincidence that increases in illnesses happens to be juxtaposed with the increase of wheat intake is too obvious to be ignored. The earlier man neither had the knowledge nor the need to feed on wheat and other grains. Then why is there a dependency on wheat products now? Why do we find it impossible to live without cereals, breads, buns, bagels, donuts and pizzas?

Through the changing times, our thought process has also been altered and we are made to believe that wheat and the various grains should be the main element of our diet. In fact, much of our wrong ideas have been fed to us through our school-based curriculum which teaches us the wrong perception of what is needed in our diet and what isn't.

We have come to believe that the most significant part of our diet is the carbohydrates gained from the various cereals and grains. And if you were to assume that processed wheat can easily be substituted with the organic and fresh produce to achieve the same results, you will still be farther away from the truth.

You see, according to Dr. Davis, when the wheat was being genetically altered, it was also the organic wheat that got in the mill. Dr. Davis has clinically proven that whether he consumed organic or processed wheat products, his blood sugar would rise abruptly indicating that the organic wheat crop also contains the same risky ingredients as its processed counterpart. So it is not about taking organic or inorganic anymore but about alternative choices altogether.

We will now discuss the foods that, according to Dr Davis, we can't eat or should omit from our diet; not only because we have wheat belly, but also because we are able to make logical and healthier eating choices in our lives.

Foods You Should Avoid

Going wheat-free would have been easier a few decades back but it seems as though the agro-businesses have personally ensured that people become addicted to wheat and its derivatives. Most of the sauces that you can think of and other processed foods are created in a way that wheat is a part of them.

Let's have a look at the foods that we CANNOT eat or must absolutely leave out of our diet if losing the wheat belly is desired or if one wants to save himself from the awful side-effects of eating wheat.

- **Wheat-Based Edible Products:** If you want to go wheat-free for a while or take it up as a permanent change in lifestyle, believe me it is much easier said than done. Wheat is not found in baked breads, buns, croissants and bagels alone. It is found in a variety of other edible products as well-and in fact once you go through the following description, you will realize that its derivatives are found in many inconspicuous places. So if you desire to choose wheat-free foods, then you will not only have to give up wheat itself (and that includes organic too) but all other forms of healthy whole grains as they have gone through serious genetic alteration as well. These include barley, rye, oats, millet, chia seed, amaranth, quinoa, etc.

You should also avoid seasonings like curry powder, taco seasoning and other seasoning mixes as they contain wheat as well. Many of the sauces, condiments and salad dressings also contain wheat and/or other starches that have to be avoided when going wheat-free. These include any of the prepared gravies that have been thickened by corn starch, malt or wheat flour, ketchup, malt vinegar, malt syrup, soy sauce, teriyaki sauce, thickened fruit fillings, nut bars, broths, soups and similarly canned soups and soup stocks as well.

Certain ice creams, like Oreo cookie or cookies and cream, also contain wheat in the form of crushed biscuits and similarly, although peanut butter might be allowed but peanut butter cookies contain flour.

Cheesecakes also have a crushed biscuit

base and therefore have to be eliminated out of the diet, even though most of the cheeses are allowed.

Now, eliminating wheat also means that we have to leave out the various breakfast cereals out of our diet too. These include all the sugary cereals, bran cereals, cornflakes (and that includes all kinds of corn flakes – frosted, honey coated, crunchy and regular), granola cereals, muesli, oat cereals (which include Cheerios, Honey Bunches of Oats, Cracklin' Oat Bran and other brands), all of the labelled 'healthy' cereals along with corn cereals and rice cereals.

Meat dishes, like breaded meats, assorted deli meats (for example salami and sausages), canned meats, burger patties (as they can contain bread crumbs in them) prepared turkey with sauce and hot dogs also contain wheat in some form and therefore has to be avoided.

Alcoholic drinks, too, contain wheat, so you know what you have to do. But besides these beverages, powdered milk and powdered chocolate produced to make milk drinks also contain wheat. You should also stay away from any other drink that mentions malt or any other sweetener.

- **Foods Containing Gluten:** Generally wheat products like pasta, noodles, cakes, cookies, pancakes and pizza breads are thought as Gluten-foods but there are other edible products containing gluten too and these have to be avoided as well. These include gnocchi, vegetable protein, wheat germ, semolina, rusk, crepes, croutons, brioche, burrito, beignets etc.

- **Fast Foods and Prepared Foods:** If you are trying to lose your wheat belly then you will have to side-step all kinds of fast foods and junk foods as well because of the amount of wastes they place in our body. These kinds of food include cake frosting, gums, corn chips, baked/fried potato chips, candy bars, tiramisu, tortilla snacks, chew mixes and ice cream. You should absolutely stay away from all kinds of prepared and processed food items too; like ready-to-eat dinners and microwave meals.

- **Prepared and Packed Nuts:** Some dried fruits and nuts are allowed when you choose to go wheat-free. However, those that have been roasted with or without seasonings and then packed with preservatives are not allowed. The most commonly sold include dry roasted peanuts, roasted and salted almonds and cashew nuts etc.

- **Sugary Items and Sweet Products:** Going wheat-free in order to lose the wheat belly also entails leaving out all kinds of sugary items and sweet products, whether or not they contain wheat or its derivatives. Such items include candies, desserts, ice cream, energy bars, fruit sorbets, fruit roll-ups, artificial sweeteners and those prepared from high-fructose corn syrups and sucrose. The prepared and bottled jams, jellies, marmalades, preserves, chutneys and ketchups are not allowed either. Other preparations containing rice starch, tapioca starch, corn starch and/or potato starch have to be avoided as well. Commercially packed fruit juices and fruits that are canned and tinned in sugary syrups also come in this category.

- **Soy Products:** Some soy products have also been genetically modified, like tofu, natto, miso, tempeh, edamame and soybeans; therefore they should also be ripped off the list of foods that are allowed.

- **Legumes:** Many of the beans and lentils should be avoided like lima beans, kidney beans, black beans, butter beans, chickpeas and lentils.

- **Fruits:** Most of the fruits won't do you any good. Fruits like mango, banana, pineapple, dates, figs and papaya have a lot of sugar content and if you are trying to lose that belly weight, you will have to lose most of the fruits too. I am **not** by any means telling you that they **have** to go, but too much of a good thing can be bad, especially on this diet.

- **Milk Products:** Most of the naturally cultured cheeses are allowed; however other prepared dairy products that are sold in the market, such as coffee drinks, milk drinks, malted milk etc. or even cottage cheese is not allowed as they might contain some form of wheat or malt derivatives.

- All permitted food colours and artificial flavourings are not allowed either and this includes even the top quality liquid food colour and the various fruit flavourings found in the baking section of the supermarket.

Wheat can easily be identified in food items like pizza, loaf of bread, doughnuts and even a box of crackers, but the hard part is identifying wheat in other unexpected products like those mentioned above. The best way to deal with such fears is to thoroughly check the food label or the ingredient list to get a better idea of what is contained in it.

Foods You Can Eat!

It is most likely for readers to believe that if they can't eat the things mentioned above then 'What should they be eating?' As unbelievable as it may sound, there are still plenty of things available in the market that one can buy and to prepare delicious meals three times a day. And if you are worried about fulfilling your nutritional requirements then don't be, because you will still be able to get loads of fibre in your body along with other vitamins and nutrients.

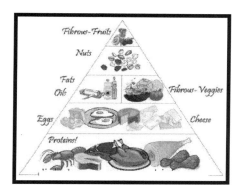

The hardest part for people who want to start a wheat-free regime is cutting out bread and buns from their life. And as discussed earlier in this book and in my other books, cutting out wheat absolutely may develop separation anxiety in them as wheat products create an 'addiction' which is hard to let go of and can be compared with other addictions easily.

According to Dr. Davis, the hardest part for people is giving up the bread and sandwiches; and this is the reason why people are still reluctant to believe in his findings even though they are backed with substantial data. Yet in his book Wheat Belly: Lose the Wheat, Lose the Weight and Find Your Path Back to Health, he has urged people to only try it out for a brief period of four weeks and the results that they experience will not let them go back to their old dieting habits; so profound is his belief that wheat is the real danger in our lives.

So then, the most probable question that falls into our laps now is 'What should we eat then?' Dr. Davis is usually surprised when people ask that because there are so many other marvellous foods in nature to be enjoyed – the 'real foods' as he refers to them. These are identified as foods that have not been changed and are grown organically like vegetables, meat, cheeses etc. The benefits of leaving out wheat and harmful fats and sugars are that weightwatchers don't have to watch the intake of calories anymore. In fact, they can eat as much as they want from the foods allowed and still be able to lose weight just by eliminating wheat and other unhealthy foods.

So basically, you will have to brainwash the old food pyramid from your mind and focus on the new one given below from now on if you want to leave these unhealthy products out of your life.

This pyramid is a rough illustration to give people an idea about what they can and cannot eat. Analyse this illustration and you will realize that there are many varieties of foods that we can still enjoy; in fact there seems to be hardly anything missing here, other than the bread of course. But apart from that, you can still have the good fats, vegetables, and your choice of healthy proteins, eggs cheeses, nuts and fruits. You really have nothing to lose if you go wheat free for a while except your weight and may be some illnesses.

So following is a list of things that you will be able to enjoy when going wheat free:

- You may eat from a huge variety of organically grown fresh vegetables like onions, shallots, carrots, leeks, chives, mushrooms, tomatoes, eggplant, chillies, radish, garlic, ginger, ladyfingers and all kinds of different herbs. As potato contains a lot of starch, you should try to stay away from it.

- For cooking and to use in the dressing, you can select from a wide variety of healthy oils and these include olive oil, almond oil, sesame oil, coconut oil, walnut oil, avocado oil, flaxseed oil, macadamia oil and cocoa butter. However, you must remember that even though they are pure and healthy oils, you should not indulge in too much deep frying or even shallow frying; also never over-heat the oils.

- You can eat nuts and seeds as much as you want. Nature has provided an ample choice so don't limit yourself. There are almonds, pistachios, walnuts, cashew nuts, pecans, hazelnuts, Brazil nuts, peanuts and then there are pumpkin seeds, sesame seeds, sunflower seeds and nut meals to chew on. Not only do they complement the dishes when cooked as part of the main course, they are also tasteful munching snacks.

- And then of course we have a wide variety of meats to choose from. You can get organic meat from practically every store now. Chicken, beef, mutton, turkey, buffalo, game birds, fish and shellfish – are allowed and don't forget you can have plenty of eggs too.

- Non-sugary and non-wheat condiments can be taken with meals like mustard, hummus, oil-based salad dressing, pesto, guacamole, mayonnaise, vinegar, tapenades, chilli sauce, salsa etc.

- The full-fat and cultured cheeses are very much allowed-. This might come as a surprise to some people because they have always been programmed to believe they should refrain from eating cheese while on various diets. Then again this is not a diet but a mere awareness that all healthy and natural food stuff do not harm the body-. It is the unnatural and artificially grown edible products that cause all the fat and toxin storage within the body and these later on lead to harmful illnesses and diseases. Yogurt and Greek yogurt can be beneficial.

- You can prepare all sorts of beverages like coffee, tea, coconut milk, almond milk, chocolate milk (with unsweetened cocoa) and even milkshakes as long as you select honey instead of a sweetener. Fresh fruit juices are also allowed, however you must limit their intake to a single serving a day. Same goes with milk too.

- Fruits can be taken in only limited quantities; however the canned and tinned fruits especially that are contained in sweet syrup should be avoided. Berries, citrus fruits and apples are more recommendable amongst others.

- Amongst the beans you can eat peas, sweet potatoes, brown rice and yams.

Yet with all these food products mentioned above the wide gap made by loss of wheat still remains in the diet and for this reason, Dr. Davis believes that you can go ahead with the non-wheat grains that include ground flaxseed and ground chia seeds.

Planning Your Meals to Be Wheat FREE!

Planning a meal with the inclusion of wheat or other starchy products could be a testing task but at the same time it is not impossible. With a little bit of knowledge and determination, it can be done easily. The first thing that you need to do is to note down the things that you are allowed to eat and then start building up your menu from there.

Of course, you will also be required to revamp your pantry and kitchen shelves. Go through all the stored food products there and the best way of doing that is by reading the labels to see what harmful ingredients are contained in them. Don't be surprised if you end up locating a lot many things that include or wheat flour.

Next, it is always better to gear yourself up with complete ammunition before stepping into warzone and this wheat-free routine will be no less than a major fight with your own self and desires. So, go to your local grocery store and educate yourself about all the things that fall into the 'healthy' category. You will find a lot of things, not already mentioned in this book. Furthermore, because a great many people are now trying to go wheat free, you will realize that there are many 'wheat-free' products that have been added to the aisles in the grocery store; for example, there is rice pasta, brown rice and wheat-free cereals that can be easily found. So in reality, you will simply be switching to other brands of food.

Once you are done making the list of ingredients that you need to switch to, you can then plan a whole menu. It would be easier to list all the breakfast dishes, lunch and dinner meal dishes separately so that you can make a shopping list for the whole week. Since some of the wheat-free products will cost more than your usual choice, it is better to write down the exact ingredients you will need for your meals so that you don't overspend and are able to save money during your shopping.

Examples of Wheat Free Recipes

In this chapter, I provide you with a few examples of wheat free recipes. This will give you an idea of what you can cook while on the diet!

Breakfast

Savoury Breakfast Casserole with Shredded Meat and Eggs

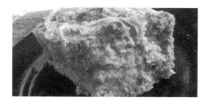

This is a breakfast dish that you can either serve to many members or you can bake it and consume it in the next couple of days. For this dish, you are going to need,

- 12 eggs
- 1 pound of meat of your choice (can be ground beef, boiled or grilled chicken)
- Salt, to taste
- Pepper, to taste,
- Prepared tomato sauce
- Shredded cheddar cheese
- 1 large onion
- 1 sweet potato shredded
- 2 tablespoon of hot sauce
- 1 teaspoon garlic powder and
- 1 teaspoon onion powder

Method

- Begin by preheating the oven to 375 degrees.

- Next, if you need to cook the meats then boil it slightly and then finish off with frying it.

- For the tomato sauce, sauté some chopped onion in a frying pan, add a bit of crushed garlic and some tomatoes. Add salt and red chilli powder and then add some water. Reduce it down, add some dried oregano leaves and take off heat when it has gotten thick.

- Now, beat the eggs in a large bowl thoroughly and once done add the rest of the ingredients, including meat but excluding the tomato sauce and the cheese.

- Grease an oven proof glass dish and pour everything into it.

- Cook in the oven for 10 minutes. Take out and spread the tomato sauce evenly also add the cheddar cheese on top. Return it to the oven immediately and leave it in there for another 10-15 minutes or until the eggs are not runny anymore. Do check from the middle before taking out.

Baked Sweet Potato-Crusted Omelette

This recipe is a slight variation of the recipe mentioned above, and it is equally delicious and fulfilling. To make this dish, you will need,

- 2 small sweet potatoes (thinly sliced)

- 8 eggs

- 1 ½ teaspoon mixed herb seasoning

- 1 finely chopped onion (sautéed)

- 1 finely chopped red pepper (sautéed)

- 2 cups thinly sliced broccoli (steamed)

- 1 teaspoon crushed garlic

- Grilled chicken strips (thinly sliced)

- ½ cup sundried tomatoes and

- ½ cheddar or cottage cheese

Method

Line two pie dishes with the sweet potato slices. Next whisk the eggs thoroughly before you add all the rest of the ingredients in it. Once you have mixed all the ingredients in the eggs, pour it over the prepared sweet potato base and put it in the oven for 30 – 35 minutes.

Lunch

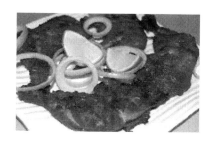

Chicken Tikka

This is a very famous Indian dish around the world and you can enjoy this in your wheat-free plan. To make this delicious recipe, you require

- 1 whole chicken cut into four quarters
- 1 ½ tablespoon of thick yogurt
- 1 teaspoon salt
- 1 teaspoon red chilli
- 1 teaspoon ground roasted cumin
- 1 teaspoon ground all-spice
- 1 tablespoon white vinegar
- 1 ½ teaspoon ginger and garlic paste
- 1 tablespoon of oil

Method

Preheat the oven on medium heat. Make the marinade in a large bowl by mixing everything together. Once the paste is ready, put the chicken pieces in it and turn them around so that they are nicely coated. Leave them covered in the refrigerator for at least 2 – 3 hours. Take an oven proof dish and place a large piece of aluminium foil. Next, place the marinated chicken on top of the foil and slightly cover with turned over foil. Place it in the oven for 35 – 40 minutes or until it is cooked through and gives a nice colour. You can serve it with assorted baked vegetables.

Delicious Grilled Trout with Tiger Prawns

This delicious wheat-free recipe is equally enjoyable for kids and adults and is extremely easy to prepare with only a few ingredients. To prepare this dish you will need,

- 2 trout or any other fish desirable (trout is an healthier option)
- 8-10 tiger prawns
- Wheat free horseradish sauce
- Salt to taste
- Black pepper to taste
- 1 tablespoon balsamic vinegar and
- 1 tablespoon olive oil

Method

To make this easy recipe, all you need to do is gut and wash the trout thoroughly and then wait for it to dry first. Now add some sharp cuts on each of its sides (make them angular so they look pretty).

Next, prepare the marinade or the flavouring mix. Start by putting olive oil in a bowl with the rest of the ingredients. When the mixture is completely prepared, then rub it on both sides of trout, making sure, the mixture reaches inside the cuts as well. Leave them in the mixture for 10 minutes only or until you nicely heat up a grilling pan. On medium heat, put the trout on the pan and let it cook from one side. Before turning over, brush some of the mixture on top once again.

In the meantime, dip the cleaned prawns in the oil mixture and then transfer them to the pan with the trout as well. Before turning brush some of the mix on the prawns as well. Cook until they are pink. Take both things out on the plate and be sure to garnish them well with lemons and sliced onions. You can serve them with sweet potato mash or brown rice.

Why You Are Not Losing Weight!

Recently I have heard and read about people who claim that they have been following the wheat-free diet and yet they are not able to lose weight as, Dr. Davis and his patients claimed on the Internet. If you are one of them too, then my first piece of advice will be not to stress over it and my second piece of advice will be to go over the following reasons and maybe one of them would be affecting the weight loss in your body.

- When Dr. Davis asserts that people should stay away from wheat if they want to lose their wheat belly or if they simply want to prevent serious illnesses and stay on the track of health, he means going cold turkey.

Then it is not about leaving out the bread and the buns, but every little single item in your pantry that might contain wheat or its derivative in some form. With this book, you will be able to get a detailed account of items you can eat and those you must absolutely stay away from. You have learnt that even sauces, thickeners and condiments may contain wheat; therefore if you hadn't cut them out of your life as yet then there presence might be affecting your weight loss. Remember that soy sauce is not allowed and it is used as a base for many other sauces so they aren't allowed either.

- Another reason why sometimes people don't lose weight is because they live in a house where other members are not a wheat-free regime and in a situation like this it often becomes very difficult or near impossible to absolutely cut out wheat from their lives. A mere tasting of "wheaty' products or even sharing the same butter knife which was used to spread butter or other spread on bread slices can also lead to the presence of wheat or its harmful components in their body. So Dr. Davis suggests that you should not even be sharing the same utensils with each other if you are the only one trying to avoid wheat.

- Some illnesses like liver disease can also prevent weight loss. In fact, when people are on some strong medications, they gain weight as a side-effect or reaction to those drugs that they are using. It is therefore advisable for everyone that before making drastic changes in their lives and eating habits, consultation with a family physician is very necessary.

There might be another simple explanation to why you haven't started losing weight as of yet, and that could be your slowed metabolism. Do you feel tired often and out of energy? If yes, then it could mean that your body has a slowed metabolism and that could be due to insufficient supply of calories. Remember, that you don't have to starve yourself if you are trying to cut down on wheat; it means that you have to replace it with other alternatives that provide you with loads of energy. Also don't try to skip out on breakfast as that is the most important meal of the day and keeps your metabolism working at a good rate.

I hope you enjoyed this book as I enjoyed putting it together for you! What's being on a diet without recipes, right? Well I highly recommend this Wheat Belly Cookbook. I think you will really enjoy what's inside, and you'll be inspired to cook wheat free and feeling amazing!

6567132R00041

Printed in Great Britain
by Amazon.co.uk, Ltd.,
Marston Gate.